WHY DO GIRLS LIE

The reasons and how to tell if your girl is lying in a relationship

BERNARD QUEENETH

INTRODUCTIONTABLE OF CONTENTS

INTRODUCTION

At some point, we may have lied without knowing it. Some people tell small lies so as not to hurt other people's feelings. For example, you might say that she's okay when she doesn't tell you what she really wants to do is bother her, but never hide her truth. It's not fun. So you need to know the telltale signs that your girl is lying. Sometimes it's easier to take things at face value than to be curious when it comes to finding out the truth...but sometimes those lies aren't trivial. Those little lies can protect you from the truth...truths that can hurt you in the end. Men can become paranoid when girls lie about anything. Is she lying because she is cheating? Is she lying because she doesn't want me to know important things?

CHAPTER ONE

Why do girls lie?

You may be the most honest person in the world, but you don't understand why girls lie, especially your girlfriend. It is never easy to accept that someone is lying to us. That's why you need to know why girls lie in the first place. Everyone has their own individual reasons, but here are some of the most common ones.

Hide the past

Many people have done things in the past that they are not proud of or are embarrassed to admit. So if your girl sleeps with a lot of guys and doesn't want you judging her, she might lie about it. Whatever it is, she may be lying to cover up what she may have done in the past.

She is doing something she shouldn't be doing

Unfortunately, many people are not completely loyal in their relationships. So she could be talking to other men or cheating on you. Even if she's loyal to you, she might drug or drink too much. She knows you are doing things that you don't admit, so she lies to you to hide it.

She doesn't want to hurt your feelings

You may not be a confident lover. If she asks if she came or if her sex was good, she might be lying if she didn't. See, she doesn't want you to make her feel bad if she doesn't have to. So she thinks it's easier and kinder to lie to make her feel better.

She believes her lies

Unfortunately, some people are chronic liars. They do it all the time. Maybe they grew up in a family that lied all the time, so it seems normal to her. When people lie all the time, they start believing their own lies. Or, at least, they want the lie to be true, and even if it isn't, they begin to believe they are telling the truth.

She doesn't want to worry about you

She may have health problems, but she doesn't want you to freak out about it. Or maybe she's dropped out of school or has financial troubles. Whatever it is, if she thinks she can handle it on her own, she may not want you to worry too much.

Be groomed

Some people have very low self-esteem and feel the need to lie about themselves and their lives in order to look good to others. Think about how many people lie on social media to make their lives look perfect. So she wants you to be proud of yourself. If she doesn't have her pride in herself, she may lie to her so that you don't lose her respect for her.

To test you

Many girls are insecure in their relationships. For this reason, she may want to test your love or loyalty. She's probably talking about breaking up with you just to see your reaction.

She may not want to do this, but she wants to upset you so that she can determine how deeply you feel for her.

CHAPTER TWO

How to Tell If Your Girl Is Lying To You

If you have a gut feeling that your girl is unfaithful to you, try looking for these signs.

Her lines sound like a rehearsal and don't sound like her at all

When I ask her how she spends her day, she says something like, "I had lunch with Ann, then I went to the mall, then I went home." All right. However, if she's more talkative than usual, this could be a warning sign. If your girlfriend tells you something suspicious, you can check to see if she's lying by asking to speak again at another time. If she retells the story exactly word for word, it may be a sign that she practiced her lines before speaking to you. Why do we need to remember what we did on the particular day those events actually happened.

Her story is inconsistent

This is for girls who haven't had time to practice their

lines. Small discrepancies can indicate that she is not completely honest. For example, when she first told her story, she said she was with Ann. But the second time, she said another friend was with her. Did she forget that another friend stopped by, or did she forget her original story? As she reflects on what she did on a particular day, she says she's fine. It's easy to forget. But when she changes her story almost completely, it can get a little weird.

She panics when you ask

After all, she's someone you care about, and if she's panicking, alarm bells should be ringing in her head. She's just asking something completely harmless, so why would she suddenly panic? You can tell she's panicking when the pitch gets high or she starts speaking very fast. Another way to tell is if she uses exaggerated hand gestures. After that, she may become fidgety or paranoid about what you ask and anxiously try to change it.

She gets mad when you ask her

This is her one of the surefire ways to tell if your girl is lying. They say things like, "I told you already!" It can be very exhausting to repeat what you have already said, albeit in her defense. Is it? Being angry or defensive when asking questions has two effects. First, she may avoid the topic because it clearly annoys her.

Second, getting angry can give her enough time to change the subject and accuse you of interfering too much in what she's doing. She anticipates these two outcomes of her, so there is no need to repeat the lie.

Too much or too little detail

With a sign that your girlfriend is lying to you, you should also be careful when she lies over texts. This depends entirely on how she usually tells you things and texts you. Some women like to mention every little detail, while others withhold the details and go straight to the point. I assume that if she's the type to go into a lot of detail and suddenly wants brevity, something might be wrong. On the other hand, when she usually speaks fairly bluntly, she can get a little weird when she starts mentioning insignificant little details.

She looks away a lot

People don't look you in the eye when you're lying. What

they usually do is look away or move their eyes from one object to another. Also, people tend to look away when they are uncomfortable. Of course, lying to a loved one is unpleasant. Therefore, looking away is someone's way of trying to divert your critical gaze so that you don't hesitate when you're lying. Now your wife won't have to keep an eye on you all the time when you're talking to her. But if she spends about 90% of the conversation looking away from her, she may need to confirm what she's saying. But if she looks into your eyes too much

She looks you straight in the eye

Have you ever felt hypnotized by your boss telling you to do something? Be careful how you get them to do what they say. This tactic also works when someone is lying. When someone looks you straight in the eye, it can be offensive and cause you to let your guard down. If your friend does this, she may be trying to convince you to believe her story. She may think that looking the other way makes her look weak and that she seems unsure of what she is saying. Makes you believe there is no reason to doubt what she is saying.

Never check again

This is her one of the easiest ways to determine if your girl is lying. You may already have it in mind that she is lying about something. I'll probably try a little fact-checking to prove she is. They try to check her phone, but she always carries it or protects it with a passcode. Assuming she guessed the correct passcode, she starts searching for messages and photos. I can only find an empty inbox and an empty photo album of her. Her cell phone is no longer an option, so test your hacking skills and check her Facebook when she's not looking. But unfortunately! Either all messages have been deleted or the password has been changed. I can't see anything on her phone and her Facebook so what other options are there? You try to ask her friends where she went but they questionably don't answer you, even online. Okay, now she's three strikes. I think it's time to talk to your girlfriend and ask her if she's hiding something from you.

CHAPTER THREE

Conclusion

Never lie to people. If you suspect your girl is lying to you, you're probably frustrated and worried. But in the end, all you can do is look for red flags. Ultimately, the liar stumbles and gets caught up in the lie. Lying can be a prelude to other harmful things your girlfriend can do to you. Look for these warning signs or use them to determine if your girl is lying. It's better to nip the problem in the bud before it gets out of hand.

www.ingramcontent.com/pod-product-compliance
Lightning Source LLC
LaVergne TN
LVHW020544160826
845677LV00015B/4196

* 9 7 9 8 3 5 2 3 4 3 8 7 6 *